"*The Virgin Diabetic* was [written by someone who] knows exactly how the disease feels. She has been there and back and has beaten it! **This is a must read for every diabetic to show you that your decisions do make a difference.** You can change your health future."

– Mark A. Myers, D.C.

"This is an inspiring story for anyone who wishes to avoid being a victim of the conventional medical model and desires individualized care. Denise writes as an advocate for health and a compassionate educator. Learn from her experiences to help solve your diabetes!"

– Kelly Simms, N.D.

"For those who feel managing diabetes can be overwhelming and an uphill battle, Mrs. Pancyrz has taken a holistic approach to help you understand how living with diabetes is not only manageable, but in this valuable resource you are given the tools to help you win the battle! She put it into a format which is easily digestible and a quick reference guide for those who want to take control of managing their diabetes. It has been a true honor collaborating on *The Virgin Diabetic* and has given me hope that as a health care community, we will win this fight against diabetes."

– Wilma Hunt-Watts, D.P.M., D.A.B.M.S.P., F.A.P.W.C.A.

The
Virgin
Diabetic

The
Virgin
Diabetic

SECOND EDITION

Reverse the Effects
of Type 2 Diabetes,
Reduce Medication,
and Improve Your
Glucose Levels

DENISE A. PANCYRZ

Dana James Publishing
Danajamespublishing@gmail.com

First printing: 2013

Edited by Madalyn Stone
Book Designed by Christy Collins, Constellation Book Services
All photographs by Eileen Laibinis

1. ISBN 978-0-9987428-0-9 (Paperback edition)
2. ISBN 978-0-9987428-1-6 (eBook edition)

www.TheVirginDiabetic.com
www.ReverseMyDiabetes.net
www.MyDiabetesConcierge.com

Dedication

I dedicate this to my younger sister, Dana; she is the person who should have written a book about illness and how to cope. She is no longer on this earth with us after her battle with leukemia. At the young age of twenty-one, she started her four-year battle with leukemia and became a diabetic due to the treatment process. Dana learned what she could about her disease and managed it with the utmost dignity and determination.

To my youngest sister and best friend, Darline, who I hope will learn to avoid diabetes altogether.

To my nephew, Chris; stepdaughters Christine and Tracy; son-in-law Patrick, and grandchildren Matthew, Casey, Dylan, and Valerie who have been supportive while subjected to my constant lectures on healthy eating and diabetes avoidance.

To my husband, Larry, who has been my biggest advocate during my new life as a diabetic. He never hesitated to say how proud he was of me while I tried to learn everything I could about diabetes. He always had the faith that I could do something good for others because of it. Without the inspiration and support from those I love, this book would not be possible.

Contents

Note from the Author

All material herein is provided for information only and may not be construed as personal medical advice. No action should be taken based solely on the contents of this information; instead, readers should consult appropriate health professionals on any matter relating to their health and well-being. The author is not a licensed medical care provider. The information is provided with the understanding that the author is not engaged in the practice of medicine. The author is not responsible for errors or omissions.

Acknowledgments

I am grateful to Dr. Wilma Hunt-Watts with whom I have had the pleasure to work during this and other related projects. Her level of care and understanding of the diabetic patient reflects my viewpoint and that of the patient. I am forever thankful of her time and expertise in contributing a chapter on diabetic foot care.

For further information on podiatric services or consultations, Dr. Hunt-Watts, aka The Sole Doc, Telemedicine Ambassador, can be reached at www.thesoledoc.com.

Preface

Denise's Diabetes Reversal Learning Methods

I experienced the dark side of diabetes, from ill health to the frustration of balancing good- tasting food that is healthy to learning how to manage doctors to working to eliminate my insulin and medication to planning and maintaining optimal health for the rest of my life.

Have you heard the saying, "Don't reinvent the wheel?" There is a lot of truth to that. After being diagnosed with diabetes, I read research articles and books nonstop. You can find thousands of articles on the Internet and videos on YouTube. With all of this available information, it can get very confusing very fast. Whom do you listen to? How do you follow this new learned information? No one is taking you by the hand and walking you through the process step-by-step to reverse the effects of type 2 diabetes...until now, until here.

I have always had a love for mentoring and teaching people. I truly believe my life's journey, combined with my skills, experience, and tenacity brought me to where I am today—a diabetes reversal coach.

Does it sound strange to have a diabetes "reversal" coach? Would you rather have a diabetes "management" coach? I think you get my point. Diabetes is not "fixed" in your doctor's office. The way I work may be different from any diabetes educator you have ever met or classes you may have attended.

I get to know my clients. We create a connection so I understand you and your lifestyle. My "Reverse My Diabetes Blueprint" is designed to get to the core of your lifestyle, to help you realize what you need to change, and most importantly, how to make the necessary changes. An overview of my blueprint is available at http://reversemydiabetes.net/services/coaching.

Learning what has sabotaged your efforts in the past, with techniques on how to overcome these saboteurs, is part of the building blocks for a lifetime of success. If you have the will, I have the way. There has been no greater joy than seeing diabetics achieve and even exceed their goals.

How do you know if you need coaching? You need coaching if:

- Your glucose is not in normal or near-normal range.
- You have tried to improve with lifestyle changes and got frustrated or bored with the food.
- You could not sustain changes in your lifestyle.
- You seem to follow more of the yo-yo diets.
- You have never been consistent.
- You don't believe that improvements or reversal is possible.
- You are unsure what sabotages your efforts.
- Your doctor believes you cannot eliminate or reduce drug dosages.

If one or more of these situations apply to you, you need a results-oriented coach. While results vary by individual, seeing improvement is *absolutely doable*.

Getting through the first year of being a diabetic seems like a long road. This disease has consumed my life. Everything I eat, everything I do, everywhere I go, I must be mindful of my disease, diabetes. When one is faced with diabetes or any disease, you have two choices: (1) Be ignorant of the disease and go about your life, taking any treatments and medications as advised; or (2) embrace it and learn all you can to manage your life and the disease to the best of your ability to maintain a healthy life; you are in charge.

I hope you can learn from the information and experiences I bring forward and understand how diabetes can truly be managed. I hunted for information even as crazy as some of the information seemed. I learned to ask questions, ask more questions, and ask even more questions. You need to ask questions of your doctors, ask questions of others with the same disease, and ask questions of others with different diseases. Be open to information to gain new perspectives. I hope my story will pave the way for you to get what you want from the medical community, friends and family, and help you lead a healthy lifestyle.

Knowledge is power; gain the knowledge.

CHAPTER 1

Life before Diabetes

When it is said that your health is everything, nothing could be more true. I made it through my first two years as an acknowledged diabetic. I say this because when my doctor warned me to exercise and eat more vegetables and legumes, I thought I had more time ahead of me to start leading a healthier lifestyle. Previously, I didn't admit I was on my way to becoming a diabetic. Many others I have spoken to or read about felt the same way. We just don't want to admit it until it's, of course, too late. When we are told we are prediabetic or diabetic, so many of us are in denial. I didn't feel differently. Maybe that's the problem—we can't see it, and we don't think we feel any effects from it. We think we can just take a pill and continue on as we have been.

A few years before my diagnosis, I found out my fasting glucose levels were on the rise. My doctor always counseled to eat healthy and exercise. Well, it goes without saying; we all know we should follow that advice. It's not as satisfying to eat healthy compared to the foods I had been eating. Making a lifestyle change when life is busy is inconvenient and difficult. In my forties, I thought I was young enough to put off a healthier lifestyle for a while longer. I was having fun in my life. If I started making changes soon, I thought I would be fine.

A year went by, and I decided to take my health seriously and improve my glucose and cholesterol levels. I ate oatmeal for breakfast, reduced the amount of fried foods I ate, reduced the amount of red wine I drank, and reduced the amount of food I ate at one sitting. I was a little better about exercising, but not consistent. Overall, I improved my lifestyle. Or so I thought.

During this time, I learned to play golf, which my husband had hounded me for twenty years to do. Chasing after a small ball for several hours did not sound like fun to me. However, after some lessons at a local park district with my sister Darline, we were hooked, ready to quit our jobs and enjoy playing golf full time! It didn't take us long to come to our senses. We did get to enjoy traveling to some wonderful places to golf—Arizona, Palm Springs, Mexico, and Hawaii, just to name a few. Of course, along with playing golf was the eating and drinking at the country club. I started drinking cold beer after playing in the heat; I had never been a beer drinker. Clearly, this lifestyle went against my earlier efforts at living healthier.

In October 2010, we were vacationing in Naples, Florida, when I became ill with what I believed was a virus. I had decided—again—to eat healthy, even while on vacation.

Did you ever reach a moment in your life when you were satisfied with a decision you've made but found out it was too late to do you any good? I did, and I call it failure.

While driving to the airport to return home, I realized my vision was blurred. I could no longer read the street signs. This was troubling to me because in December of 2009, I received Lasik treatment and had 20/20 vision. At this point, I became concerned that diabetes may be rearing its ugly head. I was aware that a vision problem is a symptom. I was afraid I had procrastinated one too many times.

Just a few days later, I had excruciating abdominal pains. After the pain became unbearable, I went to the local immediate care center. As soon as we arrived, my pain started to subside. So I had my husband bring me back home. I was hoping it was the stomach flu or maybe a gallbladder problem. (Why I would go home if it were a gallbladder problem makes no sense, but that is what I did.) As soon as we pulled up in front of our home, the pain started again; so back to the immediate care center.

I was diagnosed with gastritis (diagnosed without any lab testing) and sent home to take Aciphex for heartburn and other symptoms associated with acid reflux disease, Dicyclomine used to treat IBS (irritable bowel syndrome), and Ondansetron (Zofran) used to prevent nausea and vomiting that may be caused by surgery or by medicine to treat cancer. All of this medication didn't seem to help. It seemed odd that I would need all three medications to help gastritis. But, what did I know? I'm not a doctor.

My husband surfed the Internet to find some other way for me to get relief. He found coconut water worked to bring the stomach back to normal while providing vitamins and minerals.[1] This actually seemed to work. But, only for a while, as it was supposed to relieve symptoms of gastritis.

Something was still wrong. The next day, I called my doctor who ordered blood work, and by the following day, I was admitting myself into the emergency room. I was dehydrated and had walking pneumonia. The abdominal pain I was experiencing was due to a pancreatitis attack. Wow, is that painful! My triglycerides were 7,926; total cholesterol 776; glucose level 410; and my hemoglobin A1c was 10 percent.

With a triglyceride level of 7,926, it is difficult to know if this is an accurate reading due to *hyperlipidemia* (too much fat in the blood). A healthy triglyceride target should be below 150. A total cholesterol level of 776 reflects a propensity for heart disease because of too much plaque buildup in the arteries. It is recommended that our total cholesterol should be below 200. A glucose level of 410 is extremely high, which is referred to as *hyperglycemia*. Glucose remaining in your blood can cause many health complications and damage to blood vessels and nerves. In nondiabetic patients, the National Institutes of Health recommends a fasting blood glucose below 100mg/dL and two hours after a meal (*post prandial*), a blood glucose below 140mg/dL.[2] The hemoglobin A1c measures your average blood glucose control for the past two to three months by measuring the percentage of *glycated* hemoglobin (referred to as HbA1c or A1c) in the blood.[3] An A1c of 10.0 equates to an estimated glucose average of 240, which is way too high! (The normal range for A1c is less than 5.7)

My lifestyle had catapulted me into becoming a diabetic. I did not acknowledge it until I was admitted into the hospital with no one to blame but myself. To add insult to injury, I was also diagnosed as having *metabolic syndrome*. You have metabolic syndrome if you have three or more of the following signs:

- ✧ high blood pressure
- ✧ high fasting blood glucose
- ✧ large waist circumference
- ✧ low HDL
- ✧ high triglycerides[4]

I knew I had failed because of my lack of effort to improve my health.

I had been pretty healthy up to this point in my life. In truth, I should rephrase that and admit that I was pretty healthy up until three years before. I was like many others, getting the occasional flu along with several colds each year. Many times, they would settle into bronchitis or even sinus infections. My energy levels had not been where they needed to be; I was only in my midforties. I wasn't in too bad of shape. I was a size six when I got married and graduated to a size eight after twenty-three years of marriage. Not bad! I wasn't on any medications except the occasional vitamin or aspirin.

Over the previous two years, I had been taking a probiotic to stop stomachaches after I ate. I was just starting to take fiber to relieve diarrhea. The previous year or so, I had been eating Tums like they were candy to treat acid reflux. I was sure it was all due to aging. My dad told me, "After you turn forty, every decade that goes by, certain body parts don't work the same anymore."

I realized while writing this that so much had gotten past me. Life goes by in a blink of an eye; I never put a lot of thought behind the little health issues I was having. At the time they seemed trivial—very common problems. As I reflected on my recent past, I realized that small signs were just that: They were hints that something was not right. Our bodies tell us when something is wrong. We need to learn to listen. Ignorance is no excuse. I chose to procrastinate because I didn't want to take the time—it seemed like an inconvenience. Well, my procrastination eventually put me in the hospital. Now that is an inconvenience. My body made the choice that my mind wouldn't make.

I spent about four days in the hospital. I was told my pancreas needed to rest—no food, just the IV. A day and a half later, I was ordering food from the diabetic menu. I wondered if a pancreas really only needs one day to rest. Thank goodness I was in the wonderful care of a hospital. Somehow, the meal delivered to me was not all diabetic foods. The Jell-O was not sugar free, and the wheat bread was cheap wheat bread, which means it was basically white bread masquerading as wheat. I'm glad they are so careful in the hospital! Pardon my sarcasm.

The hospital experience was one I could have done without. The phlebotomist that came in before dawn to draw my blood did not appreciate that I was a captive audience. She rushed to draw my blood as if I was going to run away. Her technique was subpar because she did not cleanse my arm appropriately and was rough when she inserted the needle. The lancet used to draw blood so I could have my blood sugar checked bedside with a glucometer felt like a machete as it sliced my finger.

A day or so later, the diabetic nurse met with me so I could learn to give myself an insulin shot. Insulin? Why can't I just take a pill like any other diabetic I know? I did not sign up for this!

We talked about the foods I should eat: low fat, sugar-free, diet soda, vegetables, dairy, and grains, counting forty-five to sixty grams of carbohydrates per meal. I was given a little packet of information on the foods that should be on my plate and a chart on the glycemic index. The glycemic index is where food is assigned a value as to how slowly or quickly it causes your glucose level to increase. Foods classified at fifty-five or below are considered low on the glycemic index, indicating a slower increase in glucose level.[5]

It also included information indicating the blood glucose goals a diabetic should strive for. Before meals, it should be between 80-120mg/dL. Two hours after a meal, it should be less than 140mg/dL, which is the goal for a nondiabetic. The target for A1c is less than 6.5 percent. Up to this point, the only understanding I had about diabetes is that we should not eat foods with sugar. I already knew there were some health complications due to diabetes such as glaucoma and poor circulation, which could eventually lead to amputation. I understood that exercise was important for overall health but not exactly how it improves diabetes.

This became overwhelming, and I had difficulty understanding how all this information was supposed to add up. I was not getting the connection of how a diabetic should strive for blood sugar goals of a nondiabetic. No one took the time to explain any of this to me. Before I realized it, the diabetes nurse was running off to another patient.

The multitude of emotions we feel when given news of this nature is overwhelming. I was confused and angry and felt sorry for myself. I wanted to be left alone. However, I shared a room with a woman who was a recovering alcoholic. She and her family were very nice people and tried to include me during their visits. Normally, I'm a very social person, but I could not bring myself to socialize with my roommate or anyone else. I didn't want to seem ungrateful, but I really wasn't interested.

I happened to overhear a conversation between my roommate and her doctor. She wanted a liver transplant. I couldn't understand how someone who had abused her body thought she deserved a life-giving piece of another. I wondered how she could even be a candidate given her addiction history. I just rolled over in my hospital bed. I was disgusted and didn't want to hear any more.

My whole world was changing, and I was no longer in control. Doctors, nurses, and diabetic experts moved in and out of my hospital room at lightning speed. I felt as if I were in a vacuum as decisions about my life were being made for me. I was not being consulted about any aspect of how my life was going to be from that point forward. I felt as if control over my destiny had been taken away from me.

Anyone who knows me would realize this was not good. I don't like to consider myself a control freak, but I definitely like to have the ability for control when I feel I need it. (Like I said, I'm not a control freak.)

I had my packet that also included information on the variety of antidiabetic drugs and insulin, a carbohydrate guide, and a number to call for diabetes services. No one spent real quality time with me. This is the most critical period of time for a newly diagnosed diabetes patient. I'm sure the hospital network believed they had done their job—they gave me a packet. I had numbers I could call and pamphlets to read. Not only was I physically worn out, I was mentally exhausted. Thankfully, it was time for me to leave the confines of the hospital.

I was prescribed a series of medications: Crestor, a statin to lower cholesterol; Welchol, a bile acid sequestrant to prevent fats from being absorbed into the bloodstream, also to help lower cholesterol; niacin, to improve cholesterol levels; one 81mg aspirin;

Lovaza, a pharmaceutical fish oil to lower *triglycerides* (fats in your blood); Actos, an oral diabetic drug to improve glucose levels; Novolog, a fast-acting insulin; and Levemir, a basal or long-lasting insulin. I was prescribed four insulin shots per day—Novolog before each meal and Levemir at bedtime. With all of this, who has room for food?

CHAPTER 2

I Am a Diabetic

So, life as a full-fledged diabetic began. I cleaned out the pantry and cupboards and spent hours grocery shopping—frozen chicken, frozen fish, frozen veggie burgers, healthy frozen meals for lunch, frozen vegetables, wheat bread, bran cereals, sugar-free Jell-O, sugar-free ice cream, butter alternative, low-carbohydrate bagels, low-fat cream cheese, and a carton of individual-sized snack bags that contained Sun Chips, popcorn, low-fat potato chips, and pretzels. Thank goodness for Sam's Club! My pantry was now filled with low-fat food, wheat products, and sugar-free foods so I could achieve my goal of eating only forty-five to sixty carbohydrates per meal.

I was never good at consistently taking vitamins, but I became devoted to taking medications and supplements daily along with exercising two times per day. Yes, I exercised twice a day. I exercised after arriving home from work, made dinner, exercised after dinner, then spent the night reading research papers and books about diabetes. I was dedicated and felt I was doing a great job since leaving the hospital.

The weeks progressed while adjusting to a diabetic life. I was able to lose a little weight and tone up from all of my workouts. Apparently, I misunderstood when to take Novolog, the fast-acting insulin. I was taking the shot anywhere from fifteen to sixty minutes before a meal when I should have taken it directly prior to a meal. I learned, as soon as my food arrived, to leave the table to take my insulin. I hated this; going out to dinner just wasn't fun anymore.

I thought about my time in the hospital. My head was spinning from information overload, trying to take in having a chronic disease and learning how to deal with it for the rest of my life. I wondered what else I was missing.

At the end of December, I had blood work again. This time, my cholesterol was very low: total cholesterol 121, LDL 47, HDL 34. The normal range for LDL is below 130; HDL for women should be greater than 50. My triglycerides were 199 and A1c 7.5. Optimal A1c should be less than 5.7. Different sources have also indicated an A1c of 5.9 or 6.0 or less is in the normal range. It gets a bit confusing when various medical groups have differing opinions.

Because of my low cholesterol, my doctor planned to reduce the Crestor dosage in half. However, I convinced him to eliminate Crestor as I was exercising regularly and preferred that method over medication. He agreed, until my next set of tests. Funny, I wasn't sure why I believed I had any convincing to do. In the end, it was my decision. I almost gave my control to someone else once again.

I realized we never discuss cholesterol levels being too low. Our medical community seems so quick to prescribe medication. As patients, we don't give it a second thought, and therefore, follow our doctor's orders without question or clarity.

High cholesterol may not be safe for our health; however, our body needs healthy cholesterol. Reports are starting to emerge that low cholesterol is associated with cancer.[6]

I was happy to see my A1c go down from 10.0 to 7.5, reflecting an average glucose level of approximately 169. This prompted me to ask about eliminating insulin injections in the future. Based on my prognosis, he believed I would always be on insulin. He also believed I should be diagnosed between a type 1 and type 2 diabetic because my glucose levels should have improved more rapidly than they did. Go figure; I'm a type 1 ½ diabetic! I can't even fit into a normal category of an illness. I never heard of this; I had no idea what it really meant for me.

I continued to exercise and followed my new eating plan. I was very diligent about counting my carbs to make sure I never exceeded sixty grams per meal. It took me a long time to grocery shop as reading nutritional information on each product was time consuming. However, it was worth my time to ensure I followed what the doctors and diabetic nurse told me to do. Everything became all about counting carbs. It seemed like such an exact science. I had a sneaking suspicion I may not have been calculating appropriately when I included vegetables with my meal.

Checking my glucose every morning, before every meal, and at bedtime became routine along with logging all meals and glucose levels. I became concerned because my glucose levels were like a roller-coaster ride. Realizing that this is hard on the body, I needed to do something. There were times I felt shaky and quite weak after exercising. I knew I should not feel that way. In the past when I exercised, I always felt invigorated. Something was definitely wrong. To get a better understanding, I began to test before and after I exercised.

What I learned rather quickly was that my glucose level could drop anywhere from forty to one hundred points after exercising. On a number of occasions, I realized I was hypoglycemic. If left untreated, hypoglycemia can cause unconsciousness or coma. Just another thing that a diabetic needs to worry about!

This was not how I wanted or planned to live the rest of my life. Statistics show that diabetics typically lose ten years from their life span; I was beginning to understand why. With the minimal amount of information and understanding I had during this time, I was left with the feeling of walking on eggshells.

CHAPTER 3

My Diabetes Mission

I have read many diabetes blogs and spoken to many diabetics about how difficult it is to eat right. They find themselves binging on sweets and other high-carb foods. These folks are frequently reaching glucose levels of 300 to 400mg/dL.

I know several people who have had legs amputated because of diabetes, and others have shared stories of friends and family members who have succumbed to amputation. My uncle, a type 2 diabetic, became an amputee due to mismanaged diabetic care. This was real, and now it can happen to me. I really don't understand how others underestimate the consequences of improper care for diabetes. I'll gladly give up hot dogs, pizza, and bread for keeping my limbs. Getting pedicures just wouldn't be the same!

My father was a type 2 diabetic with heart disease. I know he felt the medication should have balanced out the food he ate, and I begged him to take care of his health. Extremely overweight, it was evident that some of the basic chores of daily life became difficult for him. It was very hard to watch someone you love suffer so much when it all could be prevented. As my husband and I were leaving the country for vacation, my very last comment to my father was, "Please take care of your health. We want you around for a long time." Before returning from our trip, at the age of sixty-one, my father died. It was a harsh reality that I had no control of my father's health.

We all have an inner strength, but we find excuses not to bring it out. During this period of my life, I learned that it was time to make the choice between leading a healthy lifestyle versus leading a debilitating one. It's not fair of me to burden my husband or others around me with this illness. Not only did I watch my father suffer, I also watched my sister Dana suffer. Diagnosed with leukemia, she became diabetic due to the treatment process. I could not imagine dealing with more than one deadly disease as she did. She managed it very well by making sure she learned as much as she could. Through all of it, she was a terrific wife and wonderful mother, daughter, and the best friend a sister could have. She had strength that she showed every day.

It was time to draw out that inner strength in me. Dana would expect that; she was my inspiration.

CHAPTER 4

My Quest for Help

Nearly two months have gone by. I made up my mind to be proactive and searched for medical help from a variety of sources. I first met with a certified diabetes educator (CDE) to gain additional insight to this disease and learn how to improve my managing of it. She reviewed the basic food groups and publications that provide fat, cholesterol, and carbohydrate information on foods from various restaurants, including fast-food establishments.

I expressed my desire to learn how to eliminate the need for insulin injections. The educator explained she could only teach me how to determine the amount of insulin I needed before each meal. At that time, my mealtime dosage was based on my glucose level; I was on a sliding scale. If my glucose level was between 100 and 140, I was to take four units of insulin. If my glucose level was between 141 and 180, I was to take six units of insulin, and so forth.

I broke down sobbing and explained that I was willing to do anything to stop the injections. My greatest fear was that continued insulin injections would eventually stop my body from producing its own insulin. Here was another medical professional telling me that once on insulin, it was highly unlikely that I would ever eliminate the need for it. In fact, as I aged, the amount of insulin I would need would most likely increase. I faced another brick wall, which were getting harder to scale both physically and mentally.

I was shocked to hear the educator explain that the diabetes program given by the medical community is designed to work with patients based on what the average patient is willing to do, which in many cases is not much. Even after I told the educator that my goal was unlike the others, that I was willing to do much more, I was not given any different direction or information than any other diabetic patient.

What does it take for the medical community to listen to a patient? What I thought would be an uplifting session turned out to be very disheartening. I was starting to feel like I was not being treated as an individual. It seemed like I was being placed in a certain disease category, and that was how treatment was being dispensed—by category. I wondered if I was misled by some of the literature

I read; I wondered if maybe I could *not* turn this disease around. Maybe there was too much that I still did not understand about diabetes. Frustrated and not knowing what else to do, I signed up with the educator to attend a series of diabetes classes to hopefully learn more to see the error of my ways.

Diabetes class one. There were approximately nine diabetic students in the class. We were advised from one of our handouts that we should have forty-five to sixty grams of carbohydrates at each meal (this was not news) and have fifteen to thirty-five grams of carbohydrates for snacks. We also learned about simplified carb counting, where fifteen grams of carbohydrates equates to one serving of carbohydrates. This allowed us to learn how to exchange one food group for another. Great, more math.

We learned about what diabetes is and the different oral medications and insulin that were available. Foods we were encouraged to have included one percent or skim milk; light, fruit-flavored yogurt; and a half cup of sugar-free pudding. According to the sweets and snacks portion of the presentation, we could eat the following foods on occasion when under good blood glucose control: half cup of low-fat ice cream or frozen yogurt; two small cookies or five vanilla wafers; two-inch unfrosted cake, brownie, or cupcake; one ounce or less of a salty or sweet snack item; a one hundred-calorie-pack snack; or thirty-five goldfish crackers. Who carries their ruler around when having dessert? These are crazy expectations!

We could eat an unlimited amount of nonstarchy vegetables such as asparagus, broccoli, cauliflower, celery, carrots, and so on. Remember when I mentioned earlier that I was not sure I was counting carbs correctly when I added in vegetables? What happens when you combine a lot of vegetables with other carbs? Don't they still add up?

We then have the section of additional items to select from: diet soda, light lemonade, or flavored water sweetened with aspartame or Splenda; unsweetened ice tea, and sugar-free Jell-O.

I questioned the types of foods and beverages on the list, such as diet soda and prepackaged, sugar-free foods. The information suggested eating five Triscuits and one stick of light string cheese at bedtime. Foods like goldfish crackers and Triscuits turn to sugar. This was confusing to me. We had always been taught not to eat before bedtime to avoid weight gain.

Given that excessive weight is a typical issue for diabetics, I could not understand the reason for this. This did not seem to be a plan for success. I questioned the reasoning and learned that it was to ensure we did not become hypoglycemic during the night. After thinking about what made me hypoglycemic, I knew it was the medication and insulin.

I shared what I believed was a great idea: "Why not skip the bedtime snack and lower my insulin dosage?"

To my surprise, I received a deer-in-the-headlights look with the response, "I suppose you could do that."

Many diabetic-approved foods include ingredients such as aspartame, an artificial sweetener that is created in a laboratory (commonly used in Equal). This is a substance that has been under scrutiny for many years. There are reports that it was initially denied FDA approval because it was linked to unfavorable test results involving cancer-causing agents for such diseases as leukemia, lymphoma, and liver, lung, and kidney cancers.[7] Other reports discuss how the body responds to this and other artificial sweeteners. Since the craving for sugar is not satisfied because of lowered serotonin levels, a person continues to eat sugar and sugar-like foods, which is one cause of the obesity epidemic.[8]

I did not understand why a drink like diet soda, which is not healthy, was on the approved list of diabetic foods. We were told it was about getting diabetics to reduce sugar intake, so diet soda was okay. While many studies on the use of diet soda may still be muddy, there are negative links to health. How many obese people do you know who drink diet soda? Obesity leads to many chronic diseases. So why are health organizations condoning the use of diet soda and prepackaged foods?

Katy, a diabetic girl of about nineteen years of age and heavy-set, would chat about her lack of time, so she frequently ate at fast-food restaurants. It sounded as if she was at McDonald's on a daily basis. After modifying her diet, she ordered fries but no longer super-sized them. She would then order a chicken sandwich or Quarter Pounder instead of a Big Mac or two sandwiches at a time. It was quite evident she did not understand what type of lifestyle change was needed. It reminded me of when I thought I made sufficient modifications as well.

Another woman, who was a tad older than me, wanted to know what other drugs she should ask her doctor to prescribe because it had been difficult for her to lose weight. The educator referred to the list of drugs discussed earlier in the session and suggested she follow up with her doctor. I'm not sure why anyone would want to take more medication.

There was a rather large gentleman who sounded as if he had been losing weight after he learned he was diabetic. He seemed to pay attention to what he was eating and how it affected his glucose. He mentioned that he noticed his glucose went up when he ate a banana. I love bananas. I realized I hadn't thought about their effect and knew I had more research to do.

A gentleman in a wheelchair was attending with his wife. Unfortunately, they never really spoke. I felt sorry for them. Just by looking at their faces, you could see this made their lives very difficult.

We were tested on our knowledge of diabetes, its complications, and medications. However, we did not hear much information about healthy eating during the session as I believed we should have. My idea on a healthy lifestyle was not quite the same as the medical community's. I wondered if I was the one that should realign my thought process. I still planned on attending the next session; maybe it would be better.

During the second diabetes class, we had the opportunity to watch more PowerPoint presentations about diabetes and the statistics around it. We tasted samples of some diabetic-approved, prepackaged snacks and beverages, such as Glucerna. I realized that this line of training was not for me. Safe to assume I never attended another class.

For years, I had neck issues that caused discomfort on a daily basis, so a friend suggested I visit her chiropractor. She thought he could also help me with my diabetes. My husband and I believe in chiropractic care and have been to chiropractors on and off for many years. I thought, *a chiropractor who can help with diabetes? This I have to see!*

One Saturday morning, my girlfriend and I attended a workshop conducted by her chiropractor. During the three-hour presentation, I listened to information on how good chiropractic care can help your body heal itself and how, as a society, we are overmedicated. We were told that food is a healer and could help eliminate or reduce the amount of medication that people took every day. He touched on the topic of diabetes, telling us that managing it is based on the food we eat, not the medications we take.

Chiropractic care is about adjustments to the spine or other areas of the body with the goals of correcting alignment problems, alleviating pain, improving function, and supporting the body's natural ability to heal itself. What I did not realize was that many chiropractors included coaching on exercising and how to maintain an overall healthy lifestyle into their practice.

I had to admit I was intrigued, but cautious. In my heart, I knew the course I had been on up until then was definitely not for me. I was no health guru, but I knew enough to question what I was previously hearing. The information shared that day was making more sense to me than anything else I had heard up until that point.

I signed up for a consultation and began chiropractic treatment. As I attended my appointments, I began learning about changing how I should eat. The chiropractor discussed what good nutrition really meant and suggested the type of meal plan I should follow. This meant eliminating simple carbohydrates. I was learning that this chiropractor, Dr. Myers, was concerned about overall health. He regularly holds workshops in his Wheaton, Illinois, office and even offers a recipe night for anyone interested in tasting a variety of healthy meals.

One of his staff members suggested I watch a DVD about eating raw foods. It was about a group of type 1 and type 2 diabetics who attended an Arizona ranch for diabetes management training. The group learned about eating raw, which seems true to its name. Eating raw (also called *raw foodism* or *rawism*) is the practice of eating uncooked, unprocessed, and often organic foods for most of your meals. Raw food diets may include raw fruits, vegetables, nuts, seeds (including sprouted whole grains such as gaba rice), eggs, fish, meat, and nonpasteurized/nonhomogenized dairy products (such as raw milk, raw milk cheese, and raw milk yogurt). Raw can include any diet of primarily unheated food or food cooked to a temperature between 104° F and 118° F.[9]

The focus of this guidance is to teach diabetics to eat differently by eliminating bad carbohydrates and to eat foods as close to their natural state as possible. Following the raw lifestyle in its entirety seemed a bit extreme for me, especially the thought of eating raw meat or fish, but I did learn to incorporate a portion of it into my lifestyle, which helped me to set a new course. I started with raw vegetables I like: cauliflower, broccoli, peppers, and carrots as well as seeds and nuts. I also added a few sprouts to salads.

Watching the film encouraged me to purchase a book from Dr. Myers's office, *Maximized Living Nutrition Plans: The Solution to the Dangers of Modern Nutrition*. It discusses healthy foods and offers a variety of recipes, including some raw recipes, and can be purchased on Dr. Myers's website.[10]

The book discusses real nutrition for a healthy body and mind. It explains about balancing and regulating hormones through diet that can stop, prevent, and even reverse diet-related chronic disease. Following the meal plans promotes weight loss naturally, not by counting points or carbohydrates.

During another one of his workshops, Dr. Myers spoke about shopping for healthy foods, fresh foods, and organic foods. Several attendees voiced their opinions on the cost of eating healthy, especially in regard to organic foods. He assured us it was not as expensive as we have been led to believe. None of us could understand it at the time, but we continued to listen.

Dr. Myers also shared that when he travels, he and his family will first stop at the grocery store to pick up healthy foods and snacks so as not to deviate too far from their normal healthy-eating lifestyle. Anyone who travels can tell you how difficult it can be to eat healthy. I traveled frequently, and it was difficult to be healthy when spending time in airports, hotels, or while driving on the road. It was much more convenient to go to a restaurant than grocery shop. In order to become smarter as we grow older, we should listen, learn, and just try it.

No longer taking Crestor, by late February my triglycerides increased to 244; total cholesterol increased to 202; LDL increased to 111; my HDL increased to 42, which was the only improvement in my cholesterol. At that point, I was only a week into my new meal plan from the chiropractor's office. My A1c dropped to 6.7. I'm sure this was because of taking insulin four times per day along with Actos and exercise.

Even though my cholesterol had increased, it was the chiropractor who seemed to make sense to me. After reading his book, I realized the food I had been previously eating was not getting me back to health. Mind you, I had been eating foods on lists from different hospital groups. I was becoming so aware of everything that I put in my mouth. I was eating wheat bagels; cheap, wheat bread; prepackaged snack foods; grains; potatoes, and a whole host of packaged, sugar-free foods. These were not the foods Dr. Myers was promoting.

Having recipes to work with made this true change in lifestyle easier. Thinking about the necessary changes was easy, but actually applying the changes could be difficult if you don't know where to start. We all know if we make a chicken breast or fish with a salad and vegetables that it is a healthy meal. But actually making three healthy meals a day can be a little challenging, and in the beginning, time consuming. The recipes from the book gave me a great start. To be honest, I learned to modify many of the recipes by adding more seasoning than called for, but nonetheless, a great start.

In addition to working with diabetes educators and a chiropractor, I also began to see an endocrinologist. I thought having another opinion could be beneficial and speed up my learning curve. The clinical specialty of endocrinology focuses primarily on the endocrine organs, meaning the organs whose primary function is hormone secretion. These organs include the pituitary, thyroid, adrenals, ovaries, testes, and pancreas.[11]

I explained to the endocrinologist that I did not feel better with all of the medications I was taking. The response I received was mindboggling to me: "The medicines are not supposed to make you feel better." I don't know about you, but that just does not work for me. I had been researching various supplements and asked if there was anything I could substitute to eliminate some of the medications. The response I received was certainly another eye-opener about the medical community: "We are not taught about supplements in medical school, only about pharmaceutical drugs." I was advised to find someone who understands supplements. I felt like I hit another brick wall. Going to the doctor, particularly a specialist, should be easy and helpful. Or so I thought.

She indicated that weight gain was a side effect of the diabetic drug Actos, so we agreed to reduce my dosage from 30mg to 15mg. This would allow me to lose another five to eight pounds. With that change, I was directed to increase the dosage of my bedtime insulin. It made me aware that the doctor was just balancing medications. There was never any discussion about good nutrition. This was another example of my concern on how the medical community addressed diabetes management.

The endocrinologist was able to confirm my findings that glucometers can be inaccurate by approximately ten points. I used two different glucometers, which both seemed to be about ten points higher compared to a venous blood draw. I recommend you test your glucometer for accuracy. Be sure to test it the same time you are having a venous blood draw. Do not wait until you leave the office. You may have been provided a control solution with your glucose testing kit. I still strongly suggest you compare it each time you have a venous draw.

The importance of understanding the inaccuracy of glucometers is necessary to help recognize when you are hypoglycemic. There were many occasions when my glucometer showed my glucose level in the low seventies or sixties when it should have reflected a reading ten points lower.

Remember when I mentioned I didn't feel well at times after I exercised? Having this knowledge would have helped me realize I was hypoglycemic. It can be dangerous if you remain hypoglycemic. Untreated, hypoglycemia can lead to seizure, loss of consciousness, or even death.[12] Symptoms may include:

- sweating
- nervousness or shakiness
- weakness
- extreme hunger
- slight nausea
- dizziness and headache
- blurred vision
- a fast heartbeat
- feeling anxious

These symptoms should dissipate shortly after eating food that contains sugar.[13] It has been described that when hypoglycemic, a person may appear intoxicated, and so it is important for those around us to understand these symptoms.

Based on lessons from Dr. Myers, I once again cleaned out the pantry and cupboards, this time removing all prepackaged foods. I began shopping at Trader Joe's and Whole Foods so I could purchase poultry and grass-fed beef that had not been injected with hormones or antibiotics. These are not necessarily considered organic but are a little less expensive than foods labeled as such.

Sometimes it helps to ease into new practices, even for those of us who like change. In order to keep costs down, I still shopped at a local grocer to purchase some fruits and vegetables. I gradually made changes. I learned that in order to improve my health, it was important to eat fresh foods. I bought more from the fresh fruit and vegetable section than ever before. No more buying in bulk of boxes, bags, or cans.

It was amazing. Based on my new meal plan, I no longer needed to count carbs or points or purchase expensive, prepackaged, so-called healthy, frozen meals. In May, during a follow-up consultation with Dr. Myers, we discussed the changes I made in my diet. He believed it was time to consider eliminating Actos and each mealtime insulin injection. I agreed. It was time to see if these changes were working. I was nervous and excited at the same time. This was a big step for me but one I had been asking for. This was the first person who encouraged me to eliminate insulin.

Over the course of the next few weeks, my glucose levels began to stabilize. My A1c had reduced to 6.0. Even after taking only one insulin injection at bedtime and following a healthy eating plan with exercise, my A1c improved!

Adding a new member to my health team, I began working with Dr. Kelly Simms in March of 2012, a naturopathic doctor located in Chicago, Illinois. A *naturopathic* doctor works to determine the root cause of symptoms and fix underlying imbalances, facilitating the self-healing process.[14]

Dr. Simms ran a number of tests, which included my magnesium and vitamin B12 levels. While they were within the normal range, she explained that my 5.3 magnesium level was low, optimal being 6.0. My vitamin B12 was 292, also on the low end of the scale; normal range being 200pg/mL-1100pg/mL. She explained that magnesium and vitamin B12 typically run low in diabetics and are needed to help metabolize healthy glucose levels and provide energy.

Supplementation was in order. A doctor from the traditional side of the medical community reviewed the same test results and commented that everything was within normal limits. No mention of supplementation.

I incorporated vitamin B12, chromium polynicotinate, and magnesium glycinate into my daily routine. After several weeks, I was able to see the positive effects of my morning glucose levels decreasing an average of twenty to twenty-five points. I finally found someone who understood diabetes and how vitamins and minerals work along with the appropriate diet. Sessions with Dr. Simms were the most beneficial compared to any traditional medical provider I ever worked with.

What really made my visits different was that Dr. Simms worked with me as an individual, not a patient diagnosed with a disease and put into a category. Her approach was like peeling back an onion: We took things one step at a time and gained a lot of traction. I highly recommend seeing a good naturopath.[15]

CHAPTER 5

Research and Testing

During my quest to find the right medical providers, it occurred to me I had no idea if my body was producing any insulin at all. I was especially concerned about being categorized a type "1 ½" diabetic. I understood that a type 1 diabetic does not produce insulin at all or only a very small amount.

God places us where we need to be. By working in the laboratory industry, I learned about the C-peptide test, which I asked my endocrinologist to order. A C-peptide test measures the level of this peptide in the blood, and it is generally found in amounts equal to insulin. Thus, the level of C-peptide in the blood can show how much insulin is being made by the pancreas. This is because insulin and C-peptide are linked when first made by the pancreas. Insulin helps the body use and control the amount of sugar (glucose) in the blood. Insulin allows glucose to enter body cells where it is used for energy. C-peptide does not affect the blood sugar level in the body.[16]

A C-peptide normal range, based on the laboratory where my testing is done, is 0.8 – 3.10ng/ml. The result of my test was 1.11ng/ml. This gave me hope that I could truly manage this disease appropriately even though I was *insulin resistant*. Insulin resistance is when your body has difficulty in metabolizing glucose.[17] Exercise helps to improve *insulin sensitivity*, the ability for the cells to recognize insulin to draw glucose into the cells, so I became hopeful that I could regain my health and manage my diabetes with diet and exercise alone without the use of any synthetic insulin.

Through my research, I became aware that vitamin D levels are also important in maintaining a healthy system. It may also be a component in staving off diabetes. This is important for Midwesterners and people in other geographic areas where there is limited sunshine in the winter months, although, for me, it's probably a bit late to help my diabetes. Further research has led me to understand that there is a link between vitamin D deficiency and cancer. Cancer runs in my family, too; anything I can do to reduce the possibility of getting cancer, I will do.

I still believed it was important to know my vitamin D level, so I had that test ordered, too. Normal range is 30-100mg/ml; my result was 28mg/ml. There are a variety of opinions on what a healthy vitamin D level should be; many believe greater than 50mg/ml or 65mg/ml should be maintained. Others believe too much vitamin D can have a negative impact on blood vessels to the heart. I began taking 10,000 IU daily, then reduced the amount to 5,000 IU daily for several months after which my vitamin D level increased to 52mg/ml. I again reduced my intake to one 5,000 IU capsule every other day. It appeared to be working; my vitamin D level stabilized in the low fifties. I hope this information urges you and your loved ones to check your vitamin D levels and supplement as necessary.

I also needed to gain a better understanding of the medications I was prescribed. I began investigating Lovaza, the pharmaceutical fish oil. I was prescribed a dosage of four grams per day, which seemed like a high dosage to me. After completing my research, I came to agree with what the endocrinologist told me—the traditional medical community does not understand supplementation—and I was beginning to have doubts about their understanding of pharmaceutical drugs as well.

Lovaza is an ethyl-ester-based form versus a triglyceride form of fish oil. The way each is digested in the body differs. A triglyceride form, the preferred form, is the natural state of oil from fish that is digested through the small intestine and reported to be better absorbed compared to the ethyl-ester form.

The ethyl-ester form is alcohol based and needs to be filtered by the liver, increasing the potential for side effects.[18] Lovaza may also increase LDL cholesterol levels.[19]

Based on this information, I discontinued taking Lovaza and switched to a nonphar-maceutical fish oil in triglyceride form. Only a few companies offer fish oil supplements in triglyceride form. It is indicated on the label.

Although I was no longer taking a statin, two of my doctors insisted I should, so I still wanted to understand more about it. The most common side effects of statins are:

- headache
- muscle pain
- abdominal pain
- weakness
- nausea
- liver problems
- elevated blood sugar levels

The most frightening information for a diabetic is that elevated blood sugar levels have been reported with statins. I don't understand why a diabetic would want to take this drug that can increase glucose levels when they are already hard enough to manage. The risk of skeletal muscle effects may be enhanced when Crestor is used in combination with niacin.[20] Just as a reminder, I was prescribed Crestor and niacin together after being diagnosed.

At one point, my endocrinologist advised that diabetics should maintain an LDL of less than 70 as opposed to less than 130 for a healthy person. I questioned why. I made considerable lifestyle changes by removing foods from my diet that cause inflammation. Her response? I was diabetic. I understood it to mean that the only way I would be able to achieve an LDL below 70 was to take a statin again. It seems we are being forced to manage our lives by numbers, which drives our need to take drugs. This is how pharmaceutical drugs are running our lives. As a patient, this is where common sense needs to be used. Needless to say, no statin for me.

Actos (pioglitazone) is an oral diabetic drug designed to help your body use insulin and stop your liver from producing more sugar. Actos, along with many other diabetic drugs, can cause hypoglycemia, liver problems, cause or worsen heart failure, cold-like symptoms, headache, sinus infections, muscle pain, and sore throats.[21]

If that is not bad enough, it was reported that Actos may be linked to bladder cancer and that women are at higher risk of bone fractures.[22] When I shared with the endocrinologist that I had discontinued use of this drug, she was furious that I had allowed "someone" to convince me to stop taking it. She believed the benefits outweighed the side effects.

Just days following our discussion, the FDA issued a black box warning on Actos. How is it that a medically uneducated person like me could comprehend its dangers? In fact, France suspended the use of pioglitazone (the active ingredient in Actos), and Germany has recommended not starting pioglitazone in new patients. Does this sound like something you want to sign up for? Certainly not me! How is it that other countries can see the dangers and the United States doesn't?

Throughout the summer of 2011, I maintained a healthy lifestyle, although it was a bit of a difficult time. I had an allergic reaction to something from working in the yard. It was so severe, my arm broke out in tiny blisters. Unfortunately, we could never determine the exact cause. Because of scratching my arm and then having it come in contact with my stomach and my side during sleep, the blisters spread over my body. After feeling miserable for several weeks, I finally went to a dermatologist. I was given prednisone and a pharmaceutical topical cream.

Before this, I didn't believe that taking prednisone could make you so hungry and create cravings. I was eating things like candy and cookies; I just couldn't stop, and of course I gained five pounds almost immediately. I found that one of the side effects of prednisone is high blood glucose levels, especially in patients with diabetes mellitus. My glucose levels soared to 300mg/dL. I stopped taking the prednisone earlier than prescribed. However, it took a while to get back to normal. Through that experience, I learned that the medical community had no other alternative to prednisone to offer a diabetic in that type of situation.

Weeks later, determined to work in the yard, I broke out again, but not nearly as severely. By then, I had learned how to manage it immediately by using a poison ivy wash directly after working in the yard and applying an Arnica cream purchased from my local health food store. My true lesson was to stop working in the yard.

My August lab tests reflected an improvement in my A1c to 5.9! I managed this through diet, exercise, and only my bedtime insulin. This was great progress! My HDL improved one point to 43, so I assumed the triglyceride form of fish oil was working. My LDL increased to 127, although my total cholesterol of 199 was an improvement since February, being at the high end of the normal range. My triglycerides dropped ninety-eight points to 146! It was below the maximum level of 150. This was very exciting! I believed this was an improvement due to my reducing unhealthy and unneeded carbohydrates. This was proof that we can manage our health without the need for all of the drugs.

Because my LDL was not at an optimal level, I tried a cholesterol supplement from a local compounding pharmacy. I stopped exercising to see the effect this supplement would actually have.

I slowly lost those five pounds I gained over the summer due to the prednisone. In October, we were flying off to Italy for our twenty-fifth wedding anniversary. This was an opportunity to order my first diabetic meal on a flight.

We all know airplane food is not the best, but when you are hungry, you will eat almost anything. However, the diabetic meal I was served was not a diabetic meal by my standards. My entrée was chicken with a side of white rice, a roll, and a fruit cup that included fruits I had learned not to eat, such as grapes and melon. This meal was comprised of more carbohydrates than protein and vegetables. This was just another example that many professional kitchens do not truly understand what a diabetic should be eating. Unfortunately, I was unable to run out for something else.

We stayed in Sorrento and visited areas from Naples to Amalfi, including the island of Capri. What a magnificent trip! The food in Italy was wonderful. I ate pizza, pasta, gelato—everything I should not eat and everything I had not eaten for close to a year. The food in Italy was fresh, and compared to the United States, served in smaller portions.

I felt like a hypocrite about eating healthy while on this trip. I gave in and thoroughly enjoyed myself. Ice cream is a weakness of mine. Ice cream in the United States does not come close to a good gelato in Italy. So how did I manage my diabetes? I took two injections per day with the basal insulin—one in the morning and one in the evening. Overall, I did okay for a diabetic, but my glucose levels certainly hit higher than what I was managing back at home.

Well, the proof is in the pudding. My lab tests in November were as follows: total cholesterol was 182 (improved from August); HDL was 37 (much lower than in August), LDL was 105 (improved from August). My triglycerides rose from 146 to 198, and my A1c increased from 5.9 to 6.4.

Here's what I learned: Because of my increased intake of simple (bad) carbohydrates, my triglycerides increased as well as my A1c level even with taking additional insulin. I believed that between some poor eating habits in the summer because of the prednisone and my eating habits in Italy while on vacation, my triglycerides and A1c increased. This shows me that even though I took more insulin to manage the diabetes, it did not have an overall positive effect. It also shows that managing proper triglyceride levels are truly meal driven. Medications will not save you. Eating healthy food is the answer.

It appeared the cholesterol supplement improved my total cholesterol and LDL. However, I was not sure if it lowered my HDL or if the lower HDL was due to missing several weeks of fish oil. I continued to take the supplement at a reduced dosage, then eventually stopped because of my decreased HDL level.

As of March 2012, my total cholesterol was down to 168, my triglycerides came down to 150 (borderline), and my A1c decreased to 6.1. It was again reflective of the changes I continued to make without pharmaceutical drugs, even with my poor eating habits induced by prednisone and my vacation in Italy.

My C-peptide improved to 2.89 (normal range 0.8 – 3.10ng/ml). This was great news to me, proving if caught in time, a pancreas can rebound! The endocrinologist contacted me to discuss my results. She commented she was surprised at the improvement and wondered how it happened. I had to explain that diet and exercise did the trick. I wondered why I was explaining this to a medical professional, especially one who specializes in the endocrine system. Not happy with her care, I had not been in to see her for a number of months; therefore, she was unaware I had discontinued my bedtime insulin injection, allowing me to be drug-free.

My November 2012 results reflected another remarkable improvement. My HDL of 50 was a thirteen-point improvement from November 2011! My triglycerides reduced to 90! Best of all, my A1c was 5.7! My lab report indicated "no" for metabolic syndrome!

Based on my research and testing of pharmaceutical drugs, supplements, and healthy living through exercise and improved eating habits, I was comfortable with my decision—not to be ruled by unnecessary drugs. Throughout my research and testing phase, I learned how various foods affected my glucose and lipid levels. Contrary to medical opinion, I was able to break through that brick wall by taking control and improving my health the healthy way!

CHAPTER 6

The American Drug Addiction

After a discussion with my sister on how convenient Walgreens has made it for us to obtain our prescriptions, I realized how drug dependent I became within the pharmaceutical system. I realized that so many people have been prescribed multiple medications, just as I was, so the need for pharmacies to expand services increased. Do you know anyone who takes only one pharmaceutical drug? Greg Critser is a recognized writer about medicine, science, food, and health. He is the author of the award-winning book, *Generation Rx: How Prescription Drugs Are Altering American Minds, Lives, and Bodies* (Houghton, 2005).

According to Mr. Critser, the average number of prescription drugs per person, annually, in 1993, was seven. The average number of prescription drugs per person, annually, in 2000, was eleven. The average number of prescriptions drugs per person, annually, in 2004, was twelve. In 2013, the average inched up to 12.2 per person.[23]

This makes me wonder if we are akin to drug addicts. Those with drug addictions are typically self-destructive. Those of us who are drug dependent may not realize we are slowly destroying ourselves by taking pharmaceutical drug after pharmaceutical drug after pharmaceutical drug. I wonder if we truly consider the additional health issues when multiple drugs are taken that induce the same side effects.

How many people do you know who take multiple drugs? For a time, I was one of those people. I don't understand why anyone would believe that having a prescription for drugs is safer than being a drug addict obtaining their drugs illegally. To be clear, I am referring to health issues that can be remedied by a healthy lifestyle. I believe there is a necessity for certain drugs, and I'm thankful they exist. However, I believe we have closed our eyes to what a healthy lifestyle can truly do for us.

With a car, we don't need to know how it was built in order to drive it. Members of society don't give a second thought to how our bodies work with drugs. The difference is we can trade in our car for a newer one. We have only one body. It's all we have to work with. We should have a greater interest in how we can be proactive with our health.

Let's take a look at diabetes drugs and how they are designed to work. Non-insulin drugs come in pill and injection form. Diabetic drugs can work in several ways. They

- ✧ affect your liver to produce less glucose
- ✧ increase the release of glucose
- ✧ decrease intestinal glucose absorption
- ✧ increase insulin production by the pancreas
- ✧ reduce your appetite
- ✧ increase urinary glucose excretion (working your kidneys)
- ✧ slow gastric emptying
- ✧ increase the uptake of sugar from blood to muscle and fat cells

Many drugs are combinations of the above. We take a pill or a daily injection without regard as to what it asks our body to do. Side effects from diabetic drugs can cause:

- ✧ low blood sugar
- ✧ pancreatitis (painful!)
- ✧ bone fractures
- ✧ kidney problems
- ✧ increased LDL cholesterol
- ✧ yeast infections
- ✧ muscle or joint pain
- ✧ stomach problems
- ✧ itching

And the list goes on.

Insulin comes in varying potencies. After injecting myself four times per day with insulin, I'm here to tell you, it gets old. Have you heard the term "human insulin?" It sounds safe; is it? Insulin is typically manufactured using human DNA. Unfortunately, you are not necessarily free from side effects, which include:

- low blood sugar
- weight gain
- swelling
- low potassium
- water retention in joints
- increased LDL cholesterol
- irritability
- anxiety

And this list goes on as well.

While doctors may share information with us on the side effects of a prescribed drug, I see many patients just do as they are told without question. We don't allow ourselves to completely take in the drug information to have a clear understanding of how it works and what side effects it can cause. In the case of diabetes, this is possibly because we truly don't understand the seriousness of this disease causing patients to disregard the side effects of medication.

I have spoken to many diabetics who are perfectly fine taking their medication and continuing to eat as they always have. Have you ever read the insert of your medication? You are supposed to modify your lifestyle. When you do not, eventually more medication is added, and eventually insulin. Most times, the only winner is the pharmaceutical company.

Typically, we start with *insulin resistance*. When avoiding proper health care, your pancreas continues to produce more insulin because your cells become desensitized, to the overproduction of the hormone insulin. Over time, my pancreas was overworked and became worn out. My insulin production was so minimal, I needed mealtime and bedtime insulin injections.

We know what it's like when we're tired. We may not function to our potential. Do you think the same applies to our organs? I do. Now, think about drugs that help you increase insulin production. A drug can force your pancreas to work harder. Think about how your pancreas can be affected long term.

Consider when additional drugs are added to your regimen or newer drugs that work on multiple organs. You are asking multiple organs to work harder. How long can that last?

With holistic nutrition, your body gets to heal rather than being forced to work harder. The right food choices should not make your pancreas work harder than it needs to.

I had a doctor who always told me to eat more vegetables, legumes, and exercise. The minute I became diabetic, without hesitation, the prescription changed to taking drugs. The expectation was that I was not going to make the necessary changes because I missed the opportunity before becoming a full-fledged diabetic.

Doctors prescribe medication because patients are not accountable for their health. However, the medical community needs to find other ways to reach us. Creating a drug-dependent society is not the answer.

CHAPTER 7

Step Away from Amputation

By Dr. Wilma Watts, DPM

With millions of diabetics and prediabetics being medicated, approximately 73,000 annually become amputees.[24] Even with medication, millions of diabetics poorly manage their diabetes and overall health. I believe there is no food more precious to me than my limbs.

My friend, Dr. Wilma Watts, DPM (podiatrist) is a surgeon and wound specialist. I believe the information she shares in this chapter cannot be missed.

Just because your feet are at the bottom of your body is no reason to forget them. Have you visited with a podiatrist? Podiatrists are highly qualified specialists of the lower extremities who are trained to recognize the early signs of diabetic foot disorder.

Develop a strong partnership with your podiatrist. After being diagnosed with prediabetes or diabetes, you must start looking for a medical provider who can help you keep your feet in tip-top shape. The relationship you develop with your doctor should be an open and trusted friendship from the very beginning.

I share the following information, because as a podiatrist, I have seen the pain and suffering diabetics endure from poor wound healing of the lower extremities. My mother underwent partial amputation of her foot as a result of a diabetic foot ulcer that would not heal. In an effort to save her life, the decision had to be made to amputate part of her foot to stop the spread of infection. The amputation allowed her to live another ten years, raise grandchildren, and give joy to her family, all of which would have otherwise been cut short.

I had the pleasure of treating a celebrity with a diabetic foot ulcer who traveled frequently. During the course of treatment, I witnessed how stressful daily dressing changes had become as well as finding shoes to accommodate bandages. Because of the nature of being a celebrity, my patient was constantly on their feet. Dressing professionally while in the company of superstars, the chronic foot ulcer became a daily challenge over several months, adding stress to both family and professional life. One of the keys to effective wound healing is to minimize weight-bearing activities, especially when the wound is on the bottom of the foot.

I share these stories because I want you to fall in love with your feet. It is imperative for you to learn to love and appreciate your feet by taking excellent care of them. Now that you've been diagnosed with diabetes, you and your podiatrist must work together to help you understand the signs and symptoms of potential problems to look for and how to prevent disaster.

Always protect your feet, no matter what! Developing a routine early on is your best defense. Educating yourself about the signs and symptoms of diabetes and how diabetes affects your feet will give you the ammunition you need to win the fight.

You can recruit a family member (e.g., spouse, grandchild, or child) or trusted friend to routinely look at your feet on a daily or weekly basis to help put a second pair of eyes on the situation.

If a problem does develop, do not delay in seeking medical treatment: GET HELP FAST!!! Every moment you do not address a problem with your feet, the chances of the situation worsening increases dramatically over time. Remember: Time is against you in this situation.

Make sure you have a family member, friend, or trusted partner present when discussions are taking place concerning any medical decisions about your feet. Someone who can help you understand everything that is going on with your feet should be a trusted part of your team. Identify this person early on in the process and make sure this person knows you have identified him or her as a *very important person* on your health-care team.

Diet is key on many levels. Did you know that everything that is a part of your diet affects your feet? Foods rich in vitamins A, D, and E can provide nutritional value to help your feet. Your goal is to keep your blood glucose at optimum levels. The mere fact you are reading this book says you are taking your health seriously. Bravo!

Our skin is the largest organ in our body and serves multiple functions, such as: regulating body temperature, facilitating sensation (i.e., touch, pressure, pain, cold, and heat), helping with the synthesis and production of vitamin D, protecting underlying structures from the outside world, and helping to maintain proper moisture balance. Our feet need daily moisture in proper proportions, both inside and out. Since circulation can be compromised in a diabetic, give extra attention to the skin to make sure it is adequately nourished and properly moisturized.

Diabetes affects both the vascular and nervous systems. When skin lacks moisture, the probability of skin breakdown increases. With an increased potential for skin breakdown, the probability for infection dramatically increases, thereby exposing a diabetic to increased risk for amputation.

Are your feet dried and cracked? Then there's no time to waste. Finding the right cream for your skin is something you and your podiatrist can decide. Everyone's skin is "technically" different. Finding the correct nutritional balance will help prevent skin breakdown and help protect you from developing an open wound potentially predisposing you to infection.

For my diabetic patients, I highly recommend refraining from OTC (over-the-counter) corn and callous removal products. These medicated pads can contain ingredients such as salicylic acid traditionally used to soften and break down hardened skin tissue, which has the potential to be life or limb threatening for people with diabetes.

I've had patients who lost a toe from to trying to self-heal with over-the-counter products. Some of my favorite skin care products I typically recommend are Shea or cocoa butter, alpha hydroxy foot cream (Am-Lactin), ammonium lactate cream (Lac-Hydrin), tea tree oil, and olive oil.

I usually recommend powder for people whose feet exhibit excessive moisture or what may also be called "sweaty feet." The powder helps in absorbing the excess moisture and reducing your potential for a possible case of athlete's foot. Always remember, the bacteria that causes athlete's foot likes dark, moist, warm areas, so let's keep your feet dry (but not too dry), and get some sunlight and air into those athletic shoes.

Always wear proper shoes. Sorry, ladies; wearing appropriate shoes is one of the keys to good foot health. Refraining from constrictive shoes will help you get more mileage out of your tootsies. It has been proven that wearing high heels or stilettos for prolonged periods during the day can wreak havoc on your feet as well as your skeletal system. Switching to a wider-heeled shoe, lower in height (2" and below), will give you more mileage out of your feet and cause less damage to your ankles, knees, hips, and back over the course of your lifetime.

As a podiatrist in practice for over twenty years, I've had the opportunity to witness the detrimental effects tight shoes have on both men and women's feet when they abuse their feet with poor or ill-fitting shoes over the course of a person's lifetime. While participating in an activity, the "type" of shoe should match the activity. Whether it be walking, running, athletics, or leisure, you must wear the proper shoes at all times. Always remember, comfort is key!

Checking the inside of your shoes is one of the keys to preventing foot problems. Seams, buckles, and laces can all wreak havoc on the foot of a diabetic who may be *neuropathic* or experience diminished sensation. Some of the important signs of diabetic neuropathy include: numbness or reduced ability to feel pain or temperature, a tingling or burning sensation, loss of reflexes, problems with balance, muscle weakness, or increased sensitivity to touch.

Neuropathy, or feelings of "pins and needles" in your hands and feet, is one of the symptoms one may experience when you are living with diabetes. It has been well documented that prolonged periods of elevated blood sugar can precipitate neuropathy and result in long-term nerve damage to both eyes, kidneys, and extremities, including fingers.

Discard old or worn and ill-fitting shoes because it's just not worth it. Your feet and independence are more valuable than the wrong pair of shoes.

Kudos to you, the person who is reading this chapter on diabetic foot-care tips. You have taken the first steps in the right direction to protect your feet and keep them in their best shape possible for a long time to come. Now, it's time to step into action.

CHAPTER 8

Change Is Good

Managing our health is a work in progress. To correct the years of effects from chronic disease, we should not expect to be "fixed" by drugs.

I was not the only person who realized a health benefit from a lifestyle change. After encouraging one of my friends to adapt the changes I taught her, she lost nearly thirty pounds in approximately four months. This enabled her to eliminate at least a handful of different medications and supplements.

Another friend who lost over one hundred pounds after changing her lifestyle was asked, "How long are you going to do this?"

Of course, her response, "This is a lifestyle change. It's for the rest of my life. No one ever asked me when I was eating McDonald's every other day how long I was going to do that!"

She was so right. It is so common to be unhealthy that it seems strange when people take charge of their health.

Don't get me wrong. I miss having a good old pizza now and then. However, the negative impact it has on me as a diabetic is not worth eating it. On a very, very rare occasion, I may have a slice or two with salad. I finally created a recipe for pizza that is low glycemic and tastes good.

After a while, you lose cravings for foods that are not good for you. I read about people who lost their cravings within two weeks. I wasn't quite that fortunate; it took me almost four months. Since changing my eating habits, food tastes better, and in fact, fruits taste much sweeter. Have you ever heard someone comment that the fruit we get these days just isn't as sweet as it was years ago? I do not believe that it's always a bad batch of fruit that is the problem; I believe it's the fact that we eat so much sugar every day we need more sugar to savor that sweet tooth. Many times, I just need to eat a couple of strawberries, and it quickly satisfies any sweet tooth I may have.

Anyone can change to live a healthy lifestyle and not hate it. I have made time to cook more, which is less expensive than frequently dining out. This gives me control of what we eat, how our food is cooked, and whether it's organic. We are now very conscious of the food we buy. If it's in a bag or a box, we usually don't buy it.

My husband realized after a weekend of eating out—chicken wings, ribs, french fries, and other nonhealthy foods—his body was reacting negatively to it. He immediately went back to eating healthy again. He's now one of my biggest advocates for a healthy-eating lifestyle.

I have learned to incorporate foods like flax meal into recipes, which has Omega 3s. I bake apple flax muffins, which are healthy for you while still getting a little of those bakery-style goods. I add flax meal to meatballs, meatloaf, and burgers, and no one ever knows! (Until now.) In addition to the added Omega 3s, we get a little extra fiber. Remember, the ground beef we purchase is from grass-fed animals—no hormones and no antibiotics. There are also claims that you gain the benefit of healthier fats from grass-fed cows.

Rather than cooking every night after work, I consolidate my cooking over a day or two each week. I make a large quiche or frittata so we can have breakfast ready during the week. We also love our protein shakes and green smoothies. I will have a Granny Smith apple, celery, red and green peppers with guacamole, an apple flax muffin, or homemade trail mix as a snack in between meals. These are easy snacks to throw in your purse or in the car to keep you away from fast food restaurants. They actually fill that void when you are hungry.

I broil or grill seasoned chicken breasts. Some of the chicken may be turned into a delicious chicken salad, baked chicken and broccoli, or chicken enchiladas or tacos, just to name a few dishes. Please note, no taco shells are used. We use Romaine lettuce leaves. We add fresh vegetables, fresh fruit (mixed berries or apple slices with cinnamon), and green salad for a full-rounded meal. I incorporate the raw diet into my routine by using raw vegetables in a variety of ways. I slice up cucumbers, add a little salt, and voilà, a side dish for any meal, including breakfast.

I also make a pepper salad with red, green, and orange peppers, add a little olive or grape seed oil, and oregano. Cut up raw vegetables such as celery, peppers, broccoli, or cauliflower can be served with guacamole. Doing this gives me back my old feeling of dipping, like when I ate potato chips and dip. I discovered steaming fresh vegetables gives you crisp, tasty vegetables. For years, I used frozen vegetables, which always turned out to be soggy. I think you get the idea now; just start with vegetables you like, and work from there. Use seasonings! Try ones you never used before.

Drinking my meals was never appealing to me even with products like Carnation Instant Breakfast or SlimFast, although I now make a variety of smoothies. Look for one of my recipes at www.ReverseMyDiabetes.net. If it's a berry smoothie; my sweet tooth is satisfied from the sugar in the berries, my protein is from a vegan protein mix, probiotics, and, of course, heart-healthy oils. I make my smoothie thick like a milkshake by freezing the berries, which gives me a near-ice cream experience. Yum!

I found that buying a bag of dry beans, cooking the entire bag, dividing them up in one-cup bags, and then freezing them is far less expensive and just as easy to use as canned dry beans. It's also healthier because this saves you from ingesting a whole lot of sodium. Bagged beans typically contain 0 to 25mg of sodium per serving as opposed to over 300mg or 400mg of sodium per serving when canned.

Ever wonder why you believe you are using less salt yet your blood pressure will not improve unless you take medication? I don't believe the problem for many of us stems from salting our food when it's served at the table. I believe the problem is from all of the processed foods we eat. High volumes of sodium are in fast foods and packaged foods such as cereals, lunch meats, canned foods, and frozen meals. Even those Lean Cuisines and Healthy Choice meals aren't so healthy. Packaged foods labeled "low in sodium" still contain more sodium than we should have. We bombard our bodies with these foods every day all day long. Has your doctor ever told you to stop eating packaged foods, or did he or she just write you a prescription for blood pressure medication?

Think about all of the low-fat, no-fat packaged foods on the market. One thing I learned a long time ago from a chiropractor was not to fall for this gimmick. The food manufacturers still have to give the consumer flavor in their products or they won't sell. Therefore, they add sugar, many times in the cheapest form such as high-fructose corn syrup, which will spike your glucose levels almost immediately.

During my studies in holistic nutrition, we were taught when we consume too many carbohydrates, only so much is stored as glycogen (sugar) in our body and the excess is converted to fat. Too much of either is unhealthy. Ironically, diabetics have been taught to consume low-fat or fat-free food products. Please compare a low or fat-free product to a regular product. You should see more carbohydrates in the low or fat-free product. While the additional amount of sugar may seem miniscule, it does add up with all foods you consume over time. If the food product does not have increased sugar content, check the ingredient list, it may very well include chemical-based sweeteners.

How are you feeling about low and fat-free food products now? In my mind, you probably should reevaluate consuming packaged product anyway. Look for a fresh food product you can replace it with. Then you don't have to worry about the "bad" fats, sugars, oils, and preservatives that have been added. Think about cereal. Read the ingredients in what is called a healthy cereal. Do you recognize all of the ingredient names? Even if you recognize the names, do you really know what they are and why they are added in? Cereal has become the most widespread convenience food that we feed ourselves and our children. I believe we need to rethink how we start our day.

Eating packaged food sparingly would not be so bad, but we bombard our bodies with packaged foods on a daily basis. I believe this is one of the reasons so many people become cancer patients. Packaged foods are power packed with preservatives, which I believe have cancer-causing agents. I believe years and years of ingesting this is another reason people are so unhealthy.

A friend admitted she had an unhealthy moment. She went to Cinnabon and bought four large cinnamon rolls. She ate two of the rolls then later felt physically ill. I don't mean she had a stomach ache; her muscles felt achy. Needless to say, she did not eat the other two cinnamon rolls. I was proud of her as she became more aware of the foods she ate!

I have spent most nights reading and learning what I can about good health since leaving the hospital. Diabetes has consumed my life. Admittedly, I hate being a diabetic but feel it is my duty to take accountability for my health. My husband and I married for better or for worse. It's important that we both take care of our health for the better. The strain in any relationship is immense when someone's health is jeopardized.

By eliminating the oral drugs and insulin, I no longer have hypoglycemic episodes. I no longer worry about the mounting side effects from taking multiple drugs. The biggest lesson through all of this, based on the changes I made, is that I do not need drugs to properly manage diabetes.

CHAPTER 9

The Cost of Eating Healthy

Today, I believe it's the processed foods, foods lacking the proper nutrients, and a sedentary lifestyle that pushes us into type 2 diabetes and many other illnesses. The medical community has moved to pushing drugs, and patients are moved to take them because it's easier.

The sad truth is it is not easier. It's expensive. It's hard on our pocketbooks and harder on our bodies. According to the American Diabetes Association, in 2007 the total costs associated with diagnosed diabetes in the United States was $174 billion. That's a lot of money!

Think about all the good that money could do. The organization, Feed My Starving Children, claims a single meal only costs twenty-two cents to produce. Using the $174 billion dollars could provide 790,909,090,909 meals! My point being we spend a lot of money on a disease that does not need to exist. Let's do something worthwhile with our money instead.

I mentioned earlier that many of us believe organic food is costly. What I have learned is that I no longer need to pay for medications, so that savings fills the gap on buying organic. Let's look at the following example. It may seem that we are getting more for our money when we buy a $2.99 bag of chips, a $1.99 bag of pretzels, and a $3.50 box of cookies, versus paying $7.49 per pound for organic chicken breasts. Those three items cost $8.48 compared to the $7.49 for chicken. It appears you are getting three items for a dollar more. But what are we really getting for our money?

When it comes to our health, it's not only the math we need to consider. Those three snack items contain empty calories. There are no good nutrients in those packaged foods. Some claim they are low in fat or that natural products are used. Really? Why is it when food is processed and in a bag or a box that they have a long shelf life? *Preservatives.*

When eating foods with empty calories, you become hungry much sooner than if you have a healthy snack or meal. A quarter cup of nuts can fill you up and stave off hunger longer than those chips. Think about how many servings of chips you really need to eat to feel full. Healthy fats, as in nuts, fill you up more than carbohydrates. Remember: Once your body has reached its limit on sugar, the remainder turns to unhealthy fat, adding to heart disease and impairing your glucose levels.

Healthy foods fill you up because your body is getting the nutrients you need. The result is you eat less; therefore, you buy less. This is how you can afford to buy healthy, fresh, organic foods. Like many people, in the beginning I didn't understand, but now we are experiencing the benefits of healthy eating. Our money goes to a few supplements and healthy food, not to unneeded medications I can't afford even with the help of health insurance.

Because of eating foods with the proper nutrients, I no longer need to buy Tums for heartburn. I reduced the amount of colds I contract so I save money by reducing the need to buy cold remedies, not to mention I maintain my productivity. That $7.49 for a pound of organic chicken breasts is a much bigger bang for your buck.

The other great news is that the weight will just fall off! Just look at each obese person and watch how difficult it is for that obese individual to breathe, walk, get in and out of the car, and do the littlest daily chores. I don't say this to be critical. My heart goes out to each person. Obesity puts you right on the path for diabetes, heart disease, high blood pressure, sleep apnea, back and joint problems, cancer risks, and countless other ailments.

Today there is so much talk around health care as a political issue. That's too bad. It should really be a health issue. Our health-care system in the United States is certainly broken. One way to fix it—which is very extreme and never likely to happen—is to no longer allow unhealthy foods to be manufactured. But that now becomes a political issue again because that would bring down major companies in the food industry. Maybe it would actually benefit the organic farmers.

In reality, I truly believe we should have the option to make choices. Our best choices are made when we become informed.

CHAPTER 10

Food for Thought

I would like to take this opportunity to clear up one fallacy. There really is no difference between a healthy meal plan and a diabetic meal plan. The only plan we need to consider is a healthy lifestyle.

What is a healthy meal plan? Well, I thought I understood what that was when I left the hospital.

Many of us are taught to eat whole grains, brown rice, wheat bread, and so on. It's important for diabetics to understand the impact this may have on our glucose levels when we eat these foods. For example, the craze is to eat whole wheat pasta when we may need to limit our intake of any pasta. It's important to understand that different foods impact some people differently. What works for me might not work as well for you.

A healthy lifestyle should not have a "sugar-free" or "low-fat" label on it. Vegetables should be the biggest portion of your meal and include legumes, healthy fats, and protein. Raw vegetables should be integrated into your meal plan. You can make anything taste good by using seasonings.

Bell peppers are a good source of vitamin C, thiamine, vitamin B6, beta carotene, and folic acid. So many other fresh vegetables can complement a great meal: mushrooms, zucchini, carrots. Many of these items are a great start to a wonderfully nutritious salad. For salad greens, we mix spinach and Romaine or other greens such as Swiss chard and a little fresh cilantro, but don't ruin it with unhealthy salad dressings. We make our own dressings; my husband's favorite is ranch—all healthy and fresh ingredients, no preservatives. It tastes great, and it's very easy to make.

Fresh fruit provides minerals, vitamins, fiber, and a little sweet for the sweet tooth. Berries can be a good source of fiber, potassium, magnesium, vitamin C, and vitamin K, just to name a few. Keep in mind that whole fruit is better for you than fruit juice. Fiber is lost when it's converted to juice, increasing the rate that your glucose level is impacted. Not to mention all the additives when commercially packaged juice is produced. I learned to stay away from bananas, melons, pineapples, and grapes because of the higher sugar content and *glycemic load*. In addition to understand how quickly food increases glucose level, it helps to understand how much glucose it will deliver (the glycemic load).[25] This may explain why portion size is important.

For diabetics, in particular, it is important to eat your complex carbohydrates with protein and fat. This slows the absorption rate of the carbohydrates to reduce the glucose spikes. As my husband and I live a healthy lifestyle, we feel the difference.

Because of these changes, I lost weight, my complexion is better, my digestion is much better, and my overall quality of life has certainly improved. Now in my fifties, I feel better than when I was first diagnosed with diabetes in my forties.

Let's compare the meal suggestions provided to me from the medical community when I was first diagnosed to the holistic changes I made with how I currently live:

Medical Community Recommendation

Breakfast

1-2 slices whole wheat toast

1-2 TBS natural peanut butter

8 oz. skim milk

½ banana

How I Currently Live

Breakfast

Green Smoothie—includes greens,

avocado, berries, 1/3 apple

1 hard-boiled egg

Cup of organic tea or coffee

The breakfast on the left has a diabetic starting out the day with approximately 67 grams of carbohydrates. Every item in this menu is a carbohydrate, even the peanut butter. Many diabetics struggle with high fasting-glucose levels. As a diabetic, you don't have all day to recover from the high impact of those carbohydrates because your metabolism is not working appropriately.

My current breakfast represents 18-27 grams of carbohydrates. It includes greens, which the other does not. By suggesting skim milk in the before meal, there is no fat to help keep you full. The fat helps to slow glucose spikes from the carbohydrates. Have you ever noticed there is more sugar in skim milk versus whole?

My breakfast includes avocado, a healthy fat. Therefore, your glucose level in my current breakfast will not spike and should sustain you much longer.

Medical Community Recommendation

Lunch

2 slices whole wheat bread

2 oz. lean turkey

1 slice tomato, onion, or avocado

1 small apple

100 calorie pack snack

How I Currently Live

Lunch

2-3 Asian lettuce wraps

(turkey or grassfed beef)

Raw veggies (carrots, celery, peppers)

1 small Granny Smith apple

The lunchtime meal on the left is approximately 60 grams of carbohydrates. Four slices per day of whole wheat bread is not the type of nutrition I would suggest. There are other carbohydrates/grains you can bring into your day. It can be difficult to select an appropriate whole wheat bread since most that is sold is highly processed.

I hope the example from the medical community does not lead diabetics astray believing a sandwich every day is appropriate. Additionally, a packaged snack, even at 100 calories, is typically a processed food, many times with preservatives. I don't believe we should train ourselves to have a snack on a daily basis.

Lunchmeat is very high in sodium and preservatives. Most people do not adhere to only 2 ounces, therefore increasing their sodium intake. I have lunchmeat sparingly as a lettuce wrap.

My current lunch option is approximately 15-20 grams of carbohydrates. As opposed to the medical community's suggestion, my lunch includes veggies, which are great-tasting food and easy on your glucose level.

Medical Community Suggestion

Afternoon Snack
6 oz. lite yogurt
¼ cup almonds

How I Currently Live

Afternoon Snack
¼ cup mixed nuts (without oils)

-or-

Raw veggies with/without hummus

I monitor whether I need a snack each day. Please be mindful that not all yogurt is the same. Light yogurt typically has no fat to fill you up and uses chemical-based sweeteners or includes sugar or high fructose corn syrup. Flavored yogurts or those including berries may also include sugar. I prefer plain Greek yogurt, then add my own fresh berries. My suggestion is either the nuts or the yogurt with fat, not both. The medical community snack is approximately 22 grams of carbo-hydrates and approximately 8 grams of carbohydrates with my snack.

Medical Community Suggestion

Dinner

4-6 oz. pork tenderloin

6 oz. baked potato

2 cups green beans

1 cup salad greens

1 TBS low-fat dressing

How I Currently Live

Dinner

Couple slices of pork tenderloin

1 cup green beans

½ cup mashed cauliflower au gratin

Salad greens

Extra virgin olive oil and vinegar

The dinner suggestion on the left has approximately 45 grams of carbohydrates. Keep in mind that low-fat dressing may have hidden sugar. Notice in my dinner example, I am not referring to ounces. Unless I weigh my food—which I do not—a couple of slices should do the trick.

The amount of carbohydrates in my dinner is approximately 15-20 grams. The difference between the suggestion from the medical community and the way I currently live is that I feel comfortable after eating and do not need to process the higher carbohydrates, which gives my body a break. I will feel full longer after my meal versus the medical community's suggestion.

Medical Community Suggestion

Bedtime Snack

5 Triscuits

1 stick lite string cheese

How I Currently Live

Bedtime Snack

Ice water with lime

As I mentioned earlier, I don't plan to have snacks every day, only as needed; otherwise, you can fall into a bad habit. I love the taste of lime, so that usually does the trick for me. If you prefer lemon, go for it.

Let's summarize. The recommendations from the medical community:

- ✧ Average daily carbohydrate intake is over 200 grams
- ✧ Minimal amount of vegetables in the diet
- ✧ Too many snacks for most people—may feel the need to snack from habit
- ✧ This program is what keeps a diabetic on medication and insulin. *I know, I went through this.*

The plan that worked for me:

- ✧ Average daily carbohydrate intake is approximately 45-70 grams
- ✧ Vegetables included in every meal, including breakfast
- ✧ Snack as needed, not by habit
- ✧ Food is not measured or weighed, making preparation much easier
- ✧ Improved sleep
- ✧ Increased energy
- ✧ Weight loss is maintained
- ✧ Improved digestion
- ✧ Low-glycemic foods can allow for decreasing or eliminating drugs and insulin (in my case, eliminating all drugs and insulin).

Food for thought: What is your preference?

As previously indicated, seek the advice of a professional to address your personal needs.

CHAPTER 11

A Fresh View on Life

I have limited the use of the word *diet*. The term *diet* equates to a temporary perspective on managing meals. I prefer to use the words *healthy meals* or *healthy lifestyle*.

The word *diet* has a stigma because it infers that you are not eating tasty meals and that you have to diet to lose weight. We have been led to believe this. Instead, we should believe this: *Losing weight is a byproduct of eating healthy*. It's that simple.

I can't emphasize enough the importance of monitoring your health. Yes, it takes time and effort. For a period of time, I was checking my glucose levels four to six times per day. Currently, if I eat something I haven't had before or in a long time, I test prior to eating and two hours after eating. It's the only way to understand how the foods you eat affect you. That is part of the process of fine-tuning. Eventually, the frequency of testing is unnecessary. The more you understand your body and how it is affected by outside sources, the easier life becomes. You will be amazed about your increased awareness.

Think about your overall health. Don't get sick. I know this advice sounds a bit strange. Who wants to get sick? When diabetics are sick, it can have a negative impact on glucose levels, creating that rollercoaster effect. I learned about an inexpensive remedy to reduce the length of a cold and sore throat or averting it by gargling with hydrogen per-oxide. When I felt I was being pushed to my limit, I refrained from certain activities to rest and maintain my health. I know it's difficult to say no at times, but your health depends on it. Life has moved on quite nicely, even when I had to miss a few activities.

Find support. It's important to surround yourself with individuals who support you: friends, family, and the medical community. It takes a team to make this successful. It's important to let those around you understand your goals. Write down all of your questions before you meet with your doctor, and make sure you understand the explanation you receive.

Do not let anyone sabotage your goal for achieving a healthy lifestyle. Here's a secret: Spend less time with those who cannot find a way to support you, be it friends, family, or even your doctor. Your life depends on it. If certain folks make it difficult for you when you meet to have a meal together, don't eat with them. Find something else that you can do together. *Support is key.*

It was a long and bumpy road, but I eventually felt like a normal person just living a healthy lifestyle. The mental burden of worrying how I will pay for medication in my retirement years is lifted. For someone with a chronic disease, that's huge! It lifts your spirit and gives you a sense of renewed living. *When your perspective changes, your life automatically changes.*

I'm proud to say I'm no longer a virgin diabetic.

This journey has led me to training in holistic nutrition and homeopathy. Holistic nutrition is a natural approach to developing a healthy, balanced lifestyle while taking into account the person as a whole. In holistic nutrition, it is believed that we need a certain balance of protein, vitamins, and other nutrients to help our bodies reach maximum energy levels and overall physical and emotional health.

Homeopathic remedies have worked well in our home. You won't find an aspirin bottle here. Homeopathy is a two-hundred-year-old medical system. When homeopathic medicines are prescribed correctly, they act rapidly, deeply, and curatively, stimulating the body's defenses rather than simply suppressing symptoms.[26] It appears more MDs are supporting homeopathy.

Holistic and homeopathic health views aligned with my work as a Certified Six Sigma Green

Belt. Six Sigma is a management methodology for businesses, including health care, to improve productivity by removing waste. You may ask, "Why is this relevant?" A key factor of this methodology is to look at the root of the problem and address it. Translat-ing this line of thinking toward medication for a chronic disease is the Band-Aid. Band-aiding problems avoid revealing the actual causes. That is the basis to forming my program, "Reverse My Diabetes."

Recall Dr. Sims, my naturopath? We worked step-by-step to get down to the detail of my health; it was like peeling back the layers of an onion. This perspective avoids the layering of medication.

It's not difficult to see what the problems are with type 2 diabetes and prediabetes. They are afflictions for over 115 million Americans brought on because of poor lifestyle choices and lack of understanding. My education combined with my experiences enable me to coach others to improve their lives because I learned firsthand that it's entirely possible without unnecessary drugs.

Once I understood what to do, it was not as difficult as I assumed it would be. I believe I could have eliminated the glucose rollercoaster ride if I had been truly taught to reverse the effects of diabetes from the very beginning.

This was not a miracle; anyone can achieve revers-ing the effects of diabetes. *You* can achieve reversing the effects of diabetes.

CHAPTER 12

Start the Reversal Process

Once you begin the diabetes medication protocol, what tends to happen is you believe your medication will manage the food and beverages you consume.

We hear our doctors say, "Make sure you eat right and exercise." For a diabetic patient, that gets translated to, "I can have the same food since I'm taking medication." Or, "I see my medication is working because my A1c is better." At first, it may be true; long term, not so much.

Unfortunately, many of my clients come to me already on three or more medications and even insulin. Once diagnosed with diabetes or prediabetes, it's time for a new health plan. I'm not referring to health insurance. You need to plan on how you are going to improve your health. Draw a line in the sand and determine your goal; it's time.

Has this happened to you?

Your doctor tells you your glucose level is higher than it was on your last visit. You need to change your diet or you will be put on medication.

You make small modifications, but the improvements don't last long.

You fill your prescription, and your glucose levels improve.

Over time, you're frustrated because the medication doesn't seem to work anymore.

After your next visit, your dosage is increased; eventually, another medication is added.

You start to worry about drug side effects.

Welcome to the diabetes roller-coaster ride.

I learned, as a diabetic, to think outside of the conventional health care box:

Understand the effects of your disease.

Understand how your medication works, how it makes your body work and react.

Understand your lab tests.

Be clear that minor changes may not be enough.

Be ready to improve and reverse the effects of your diabetes no matter what it takes.

Realize you are the leader of your health; everyone else is just a team member. Yes, that includes your physician.

If your doctor is not working for you, find one who will.

Chart your plan to achieve your goals:

- ✧ Evaluate your physician. It's time to decide to keep him or her or find a new one.
- ✧ Review your lab results:
  - ✧ Fasting glucose
  - ✧ A1c
- ✧ Evaluate your lifestyle. Be honest with yourself. Do you need to add in more time to exercise? Plan for fifteen minutes each day. Are you willing to change your eating and drinking habits?
- ✧ Be willing to test your glucose daily.
- ✧ Determine your goals and set a time line. Keep it realistic. Discuss it with your physician or coach.

If you are near optimal levels, it may not take too long to see optimal results. If you are far away from normal levels, give yourself more time. Big reminder here: *This new attitude is for the rest of your life.*

Start with the following five steps to begin reversing the effects of your diabetes. These five steps need to be followed closely:

1. Eliminate fast food, including those seem-

ingly healthy picks like chicken and salads. They are high in sodium and other unknown ingredients because of processing. Limit any restaurant-type food and beverage. Sorry to say, ditch the caramel macchiato and frappes, even those so-called energy drinks.

2. Foods that come in a bag or box, throw them out now! Set your foundation for success. Foods like dried beans are, of course, fine. Canned soups, crackers, pretzels, cookies; we all know bread is a no-no, and even your breakfast cereal should go!

3. Think *nutrition*, not *diet*. We know diets do not work long term. *Diets* make us think of being restricted from our favorite foods. Flip the switch to think about good nutrition, whole foods that provide us the nutrients we need. Remove yourself from the carb-overload era we live in today, and let your body start to heal now. Amazing things will happen!

4. It takes teamwork to reverse your diabetes. Work with your doctor; tell him or her your health goals. Or, find a doctor who will work with you if your current one won't. Let your family and friends know how they can support you.

5. Exercise. Walking is a good start. Try to get in a little weight training; it's great for insulin resistance. The body was not designed to be a couch potato—let's move!

People ask me time and again, "Which diet do you follow?" I suggest you follow what your body tells you. Some people feel better on a vegetarian or vegan diet, some with animal protein, some with more complex carbohydrates. Some people have difficulty with dairy, others do not.

For me, I feel I have more variety when I choose to select food based on nutrition rather than a specific diet. I'm following what works for me, not a rule of diet. That is how I manage the psychological aspect of keeping the lifestyle changes I have made. This mind-set keeps me thinking of *nutrition*, not *diet*.

I have learned a few things over the years, be it personally through managing employees or as a consultant. When you want to accomplish something, stop the notion that you need to do it all by yourself. Success in meeting your goal is having the right team surrounding you. When your health or the health of your family is at stake, it's the most important goal you will ever have to achieve.

Don't let high glucose levels keep you down. If you need help, please contact me for your free consultation:

Visit: www.ReverseMyDiabetes.net

E-mail: Info@ReverseMyDiabetes.net

I wish you the best of health!

P.S. Look for recipes at the end of this book.

Recipes

Plain Donuts

3/4 cup almond flour, sifted

1/4 cup coconut flour, sifted

1/2 cup Xylitol

1 tsp baking powder (aluminum free)

1/4 tsp salt

1/4 tsp ground nutmeg*

1/8 tsp cinnamon

1 ½ tsp real vanilla

1/3 cup organic sour cream

3 organic eggs

1 tablespoon organic butter, melted

*If you're not a nutmeg lover, cut back to 1/8 tsp.

Use 6 or 12 count donut pan. Prepare donut pan with virgin coconut oil.

Preheat oven to 425°F.

In large bowl, stir together flour, Xylitol, baking powder, salt, cinnamon, and nutmeg. Add sour cream, eggs and butter; stir until just combined. Fill each doughnut cup approximately 1/2 full with 1 tablespoon of batter. Spread batter around center post to edges of cup.

Bake approximately 12 minutes or until a toothpick comes out clean.

Cool in pan 3 minutes; remove to cooling grid. Donuts are best served fresh.

Makes about 12 mini doughnuts or 6 larger.

NOTE: Remember, even though this is a low-glycemic donut, it's still a donut. Wrap and freeze for later.

Cinnamon Smoothie

Handful of Kale (organic)
Handful of Spinach (organic)
Cinnamon to taste
½ Granny Smith apple (organic)
Lemon slice
Water
Ice

Add all ingredients (except lemon) in a Nutri-bullet/Ninja individual size cup, or other similar processor.

Squeeze in lemon. Push the Start button and liquefy!

NOTE: Adjust amount of all ingredients to taste. Smoothies can be nutritious or a carb-overload beverage. Many smoothie recipes have too much sugar, even with fresh fruit.

Access to additional recipes, will be available in my workbook, *Reverse My Diabetes Guide: Step-by-Step Actions for Success,* and through my eLearning program, *My Diabetes Concierge™* at www.MyDiabetesConcierge.com.

Recipes have been tested and approved by clients, friends and family. Bon appétit!

Notes

1. "Gastritis Symptoms," Himalaya Home Remedies, accessed January 5, 2013, http://www.himalayahomeremedies.com/homeremedies_gastritis.htm

2. "Diagnosis of Diabetes and Prediabetes," National Institutes of Health, accessed January 10, 2017, http://diabetes.niddk.nih.gov/dm/pubs/diagnosis/diagnosis_508.pdf

3. "A1c", American Diabetes Association, accessed January 5, 2013, http://www.diabetes.org/living-with-diabetes/treatment-and-care/blood-glucose-control/a1c/

4. "Metabolic Syndrome," National Institutes of Health, accessed January 5, 2013, http://www.ncbi.nlm.nih.gov/pubmedhealth/PMH0004546/

5. "Glycemic index and glycemic load for 100+ foods", Harvard Health Publications, accessed March 11, 2017, http://www.health.harvard.edu/diseases-and-conditions/glycemic_index_and_glycemic_load_for_100_foods

6. NIH.gov, "Understanding cholesterol: his is bad but too low may also be risky – is low cholesterol associated with cancer?", accessed February 18, 2017, http://ncbi.nlim.nih.gov/pubmed/24601696

7. "Courageous FDA Whistleblower Jerome Bressler Died," World National Health Organization, accessed January 5, 2013, http://www.wnho.net/courageous_fda_whistleblower_j_bressler_died.htm

8. "Artificial Sweeteners: More Sour than You Ever Imagined," Joseph Mercola, D.O., accessed January 5, 2013, http://www.mercola.com/Downloads/bonus/aspartame/report.aspx

9. "Raw Food Diet: What Should I Know?" About .com, accessed January 5, 2013, http://altmedicine.about.com/od/popularhealthdiets/a/Raw_Food.htm

10. Dr. Mark Myers, accessed January 5, 2013, http://www.wheatonchiropractic.com/

11. "Endocrinology," last modified December 31, 2102, http://en.wikipedia.org/wiki/Endocrinology

12. "Hypoglycemia", MayClinic.org, accessed March 11, 2017, http://www.mayoclinic.org/diseases-conditions/hypoglycemia/basics/complications/con-20021103

13. "Symptoms of Low Blood Sugar," WebMD, January 6, 2013, http://www.webmd.com/a-to-z-guides/symptoms-of-low-blood-sugar-topic-overview

14. "Definition of Naturopathic Medicine", AANP, accessed March 11, 2017, http:// http://www.naturopathic.org/content.asp?contentid=59

15. "Online Directory", AANP, accessed March 11, 2017, http://www.naturopathic.org/AF_MemberDirectory.asp?version=2

16. "C-Peptide," WebMD, accessed January 9, 2017, http://diabetes.webmd.com/c-peptide

17. "Insulin Sensitivity", Diabetes.co.uk, accessed March 11, 2017, http://www.diabetes.co.uk/insulin-sensitivity.html

18. "Fish Oil Triglycerides vs. Ethyl Esters," Physician Recommended Nutriceuticals, accessed January 9, 2017, http://www.prnomegahealth.com/wp-content/uploads/TGvsEE_English_04-05-11_review2.pdf

19. "Patient Information Leaflet," *Lovaza*, accessed January 14, 2013, http://us.gsk.com/products/assets/us_lovaza.pdf

20. "Important Information for Patients," *Crestor*, accessed January 14, 2013, http://www.crestor.com/c/explore-crestor/side-effects.aspx

21. "Important Safety Information," Takeda Pharmaceuticals, accessed January 14, 2013, http://general.takedapharm.com/Actos/ActosISI.html

22. Ibid

23. "Prescription Drug Use and Spending on the Rise", PharmacyTimes.com, accessed January 9, 2017, http://www.pharmacytimes.com/news/prescription-drug-use-and-spending-on-the-rise, April 15, 2014

24. "Statistics About Diabetes," American Diabetes Association, accessed November 11, 2016, http://www.diabetes.org/diabetes-basics/statistics/

25. "Glycemic index and glycemic load for 100+ foods", Harvard Health Publications, accessed March 11, 2017, http://www.health.harvard.edu/diseases-and-conditions/glycemic_index_and_glycemic_load_for_100_foods

26. Stephen Cummings, MD and Dana Ullman, MPH, *Everybody's Guide to Homeopathic Medicines,* Third Edition, (New York: Penguin, 2004)

About the Author

Denise A. Pancyrz has two beautiful stepdaughters and four adorable grandchildren. She was born and raised in the Chicago area, where she lived for fifty years. Denise and her husband uprooted themselves to relocate in Southwest Florida for sunshine, beaches, and palm trees.

It was her family and friends who supported her through her life-changing experience. Believing that God puts us where we need to be, Denise spent a decade in the laboratory industry as a Certified Six Sigma Green Belt, unknowingly preparing her for a journey she never planned for. When life hands you lemons, you make lemonade. This became Denise's driving force to coach others to reverse the effects of diabetes.

Denise continues to keep her diabetes at bay through a healthy lifestyle, never regretting one moment. This is her life's work, to bring awareness about diabetes, a disease she believes shouldn't exist.

Contributing her time on the Retail Food Committee and Co-Chair on the Steering and Leadership Team for the Blue Zones Project®–Southwest Florida, a way to bring the community into the fold of making healthy lifestyle changes.

Denise continues to write books, blogs, and eLearning programs, is a trainer and motivational speaker for groups and companies, and conducts private and group coaching.

Some of her publications include:

Reverse My Diabetes Guide: Step-by-Step Actions for Success, a workbook that takes you by the hand to help you sidestep and overcome challenges that can sabotage your efforts.

My Diabetes Concierge™, an eLearning program available 24/7 from your PC, iPad, or phone. Through videos, audio, and articles, this program takes you step-by-step to reverse the effects of diabetes, just like Denise did; it can be found at: www. MyDiabetesConcierge.com.

The guide book and eLearning program are a complement to each other. They can be used on their own or together.

Denise urges you to post on her Facebook or Twitter page. She loves to hear her readers' stories, so let her know how you're doing!

"Share handy tips and ideas that keep you going. The more we all share, the better opportunity we have to receive the appropriate help."

Facebook:

http://www.facebook.com/reversemydiabetes

Twitter:

http://www.twitter.com/mydiabetesgone